with ease

with ease

NAVIGATING THE
MEDICAL OFFICE VISIT

Elita Wyckoff-Jones, MD

Shamolie Wyckoff, MD

SEW light, LLC
Atlanta, GA

The Content of this book provides helpful information and discussions about how to prepare for, what to expect, and how to make the most of, routine office visits with your physician, trips to an urgent care facility or a hospital and other related subjects. The information and other content contained in this Book are not intended to, and should not be construed as, medical advice. The information in this book is no substitute for professional medical expertise or treatment.

This book is not meant to be used, nor should it be used, to diagnose or treat any medical condition. For diagnosis or treatment of any health or medical concern, consult a physician. If you or any other person close to you has a medical concern or problem, you should consult with your health care provider or seek other professional medical treatment. Never disregard professional medical advice or delay in seeking it because of something that you have read in this book. If you think you may have a medical emergency, call your doctor or emergency services immediately.

The opinions and views expressed in this book are those of the authors and are not related to and have no affiliation with any hospital, health care practice, academic or other institution.

ISBN: 978-1-7356909-0-2 - Paperback

Library of Congress Control Number: 2020921810

Printed in the United States of America   1 1 0 4 2 0

This paper meets the requirements of ANSI/NISO Z39.48-1992 (Permanence of Paper)

All photography © 2020 John Stephens/JAS Photo

*To those that poured into me knowledge, joy, confidence,
and the will to persevere. It is for you that I empower
others. And it is for my daughters, Sydney and Sage that
I continue to strive for the best version of me.*

Elita

*To my parents, James and Shelley Wyckoff. They have
planted and nurtured generosity, vision without
boundaries and strength in me. They serve as living
examples of unflinching love, dedication and resilience.*

Shamolie

CONTENTS

PREFACE

Elita

As a young girl growing up in Alabama, the dream of being a doctor seemed more like a box to check than an impossible, extraordinary feat that few accomplish. Despite the apparent odds, I simply took one step at a time: Make all A's in high school. Get a scholarship to a good college. Graduate from said college with admission to medical school. Along the way, jump, climb and traverse each obstacle from prejudice, lack of resources, and loneliness, to poor performance. My mantra remained the same: Persevere.

So what happens after you've checked all the boxes and start living life? Some, like me, create new boxes to check. I'm a wife, mother, doctor and an inconsistent community servant. Now, that last box is checked sometimes but not all the time. Time and energy allotted for volunteer work, community activism, and empowering the underserved is elusive at best.

But, an idea formed after countless questions from family and friends about the best way to communicate with their doctors. I had an idea, more like an epiphany. My sister and I explored ways to contribute to the culture, the community, and the uninformed. The idea seemed simple enough:

Let's share what we know about medicine.

No, not actual medicine or textbook information, but how to navigate medicine and maximize its benefits to each person. It's not that medicine has secrets. But just like any other area, insider information is the best kind of information. It could be a joint effort with different perspectives from varying specialities in medicine from women with expansive experiences in medicine. The two of us graduated from medical school in different regions of the country and traveled to different continents for medical mission work, and developed relationships with people spanning various and often opposing economic, social, religious and political perspectives.

We wrote this to guide, educate, create dialogue, and open doors for those seeking improved health maintenance and self-awareness in medicine. Each person—regardless of education, economic class, first language, gender or community standing—should be equipped with the opportunity to enhance and maximize their interaction and experience in a medical office visit.

Shamolie

Aspirations and Joy. Expectations and Anxiety. Setbacks and Disappointments. Perseverance unfolding into Blessings. These experiences and feelings cycling throughout my life would be the driving force propelling me forward. Forward past the acres of cotton fields I would pass by on my way to high school, until the day I raised my hand during the initiating white coat ceremony pledging myself to a career in the field of medicine.

The granddaughter of coal miner and steel mill workers, I knew that I would need the same tenacity as my grandfathers to stay the course on the road to becoming a physician. In medical school, I expected difficulty and expected to endure grueling hours of study, mounds upon mounds of information, and formidable supervising attending physicians, to name a few of the many obstacles to overcome.

Over the years, I came to understand that the true challenge laid outside the textbooks, board exams, and lectures. It lay in navigating an imperfect system rooted in the legacy of medical mistrust and unconscious bias.

There are unfortunately many factors in medicine that may have led to the emergence of a growing patient consensus of mistrust, helplessness, disappointment and frustration when interacting with our health care system, its front line workers, and the background players. But this does not have to be the norm. Good relationships can occur within healthcare, allowing medical providers to competently assist and guide you through injuries, illness and setbacks.

Our unique American health care system may not be known for being the most streamlined or practical, since it can have detours, alternate routes, and complicated maps and directions. However, in doctor-patient interactions, there is an abundance of opportunities to comfort, strengthen, inform and provide hope.

For many, the misnomer "healthcare for all" is only as inclusive as one's opportunities, information, access, resources and circumstances. But with the right understanding and the right tools, anyone can begin to impact their own healthcare and get on the highway to better health outcomes.

My sister and I wrote this book to offer assistance in getting the most out your healthcare visit through knowledge and preparation. Use it as a resource. Each chapter takes you through ways to minimize the chance for miscommunication and misinformation. These opportunities can involve the choice of the words you use or what you do before even walking through the door. We are simply attempting to help remove barriers to your achieving a more trusting relationship with your medical provider and a better healthcare encounter overall.

We invite you to no longer be a passenger, but to be in the driver's seat of your healthcare experience. My hope is that, after you read this guide, when it comes to your healthcare the road signs will be clear, you avoid potholes, and you arrive at your destination with ease.

CHAPTER 1

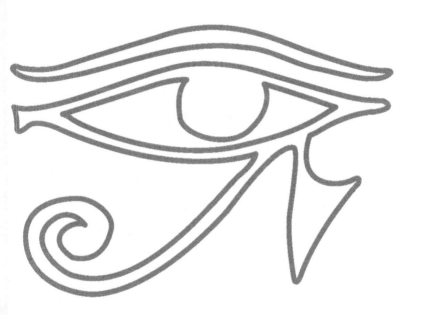

Know Your
Medical Provider

1

"Am I seeing a doctor today?"

When most people think of a health care provider, they automatically think of a doctor. This thought is instilled from decades of associating medical care with doctors. Historians have fully documented the role of physicians, yet midwives and nurses have been depicted less frequent. But in today's culture, mid-level (i.e., non-physician) medical providers hold a more prominent role in patient care. Along with many shifts in healthcare, insurance coverage and medical culture, the ratio of physicians to patient population has declined. According to the U.S. census, at the end of 2016, a total of

953,695 actively licensed physicians in the United States were serving a national population of 323 million people. This translates to 338 individuals per doctor. Therefore the need for non-physician providers to bridge the gap in healthcare has developed, and an increase in mid-level providers such as physician assistants, nurse practitioners, and midwives has ensued.

One benefit of the growing number of mid-level providers is that it has increased access to healthcare. Mid-level providers can be found in every state, in every level of care, and within every specialty making these skilled professionals essential to the health care system. Today, mid-levels such as nurse practitioners and physician assistants take on many of the services and roles that were traditionally provided by doctors. So, let's begin with defining who medical providers are, because that is key to navigating and optimizing each medical visit.

A *physician* is a doctor of medicine. This person

uses medicine to treat injuries, illness, and disease processes for the purpose of improving a patient's health. A physician earns a doctoral degree in medicine only after completing medical or osteopathic school and going through several additional years of training through a hospital-based residency training program in their selected specialty. To place the letters MD or DO after their names, doctors are also required to pass a tedious licensing examination.

More specifically, there are doctors of allopathic medicine (MDs) and doctors of osteopathic medicine (DOs). MDs are trained to focus on the diagnosis and treatment of disease with treatments such as drugs and surgery whereas DOs are trained to utilize a whole-body approach that encompasses manual medical therapies.

A *physician's assistant,* often known as a PA, is a mid-level provider who works closely with physicians. Physician assistants function much like doctors. They examine patients, diagnose diseases,

4

prescribe medicines, and write referrals to specialists. However, these professionals must work under a medical doctor's supervision. PAs are educated at the master's degree level and are trained to practice medicine using a curriculum modeled on medical school education. A PA program usually lasts 26 to 27 months, plus additional clinical hours. This differs from Nurse Practitioners (NPs) who are trained in the advanced practice of nursing.

A *registered nurse* is known as a RN. This provider typically holds a bachelor's degree in nursing or—at a minimum—an associate's degree in nursing. Passing a state's certification exam is required for licensure. Though with a more limited scope than physicians, nurses are trained to care for patients in a variety of settings such as hospitals, outpatient centers, surgical facilities, etc. Within these settings, they play an integral role in management of medications and infection control, and provide care and comfort to patients.

Licensed practical nurses, or LPNs, are often confused with RNs, but their jobs are actually very different. LPNs report to RNs and perform more entry-level duties such as taking vital signs, assisting with tests, administering medication, filling out medical records, and helping patients with daily activities like eating and getting dressed. Their scope of practice is due to their more limited educational requirement, which typically requires one year of coursework after high school and state licensure.

RNs are patient advocates driving health education and maintenance, identifying risk potential, and supporting psycho-social health. They are not required to specialize, and many choose to be generalists. However, some nurses specialize by undergoing further experience, clinical practice, and education in a specialized field. Some nurses have obtained a master's of science in nursing or a doctorate of nursing practice. Nurses who obtain such advanced degrees or certification are called ***advanced*** *practice registered nurses (APRNs).* Nurse anesthetists (CRNAs), nurse practitioners (NPs), and certified nurse midwives (CNMs) are all APRNs. Of note, APRNs have more independence and, within limits, have more freedom to act without the supervision of a physician. Ultimately they provide a higher level of care than a registered nurse.

The most commonly encountered APRNs are *nurse practitioners* (NPs) who also are considered mid-level providers. Like PAs, NPs are educated at the master's degree level but can also get their doctorate of nursing practice. Their training allows for them to order, perform and interpret diagnostic tests such as radiology imaging and lab work. They can manage overall medical care, can diagnose and treat acute and chronic conditions, and can perform certain medical procedures. Educating and counseling patients is also a routine part of a NP's job. Because nursing regulations vary from state to state, in some states NPs can practice on their own without the supervision of a doctor, while in other states NPs must work under a supervising physician in order to prescribe medications.

A *medical assistant* (MA) is a person hired to assist a provider in retrieving vital medical information from a patient. At a minimum, the MA usually has completed a certificate of training. Daily duties may include recording medical information and test results, conducting patient interviews, taking and recording vital signs, collecting specimens, and administering medications under a physician's supervision. Certified medical assistants work in physicians' offices, clinics, or other healthcare facilities. Their job often involves effectively communicating with patients and relaying that information to the provider.

Key Points

- Know and understand what type of medical provider is taking care of you.

- You may not see a doctor, but instead a mid-level provider.

- Mid-level providers include physician assistants, certified nursing midwives, nurse practitioners, and other advanced practice registered nurses (APRNs).

Acronyms

MD: Doctor of Medicine An allopathic physician; a doctor trained in the use of medications or surgery to treat disease.

DO: Doctor of Osteopathic Medicine An osteopathic physician; a doctor trained to utilize a whole-body approach that encompasses manual medical therapies.

PA: Physician's Assistant A provider with a master's degree level of education, who works closely with a patient's principal healthcare provider.

CRNA: Certified Nurse Anesthetist An advanced practice RN who administers anesthesia for patients undergoing surgery or other medical procedures.

CNS: Clinical Nurse Specialist An advanced practice RN who provides leadership and high-level clinical expertise in a specialty area of medicine (for example, in community health or geriatrics).

CNM: Certified Nurse Midwife An advanced practice RN who specializes in the care of women throughout pregnancy, delivery, and the postpartum period.

NP: Nurse Practitioner An advanced practice RN who provides comprehensive care to patients and who in some states can prescribe medications.

Primary Care Physicians *typically practice in:*

- *Internal and General Practice Medicine*
- *Family Medicine*
- *Pediatrics*
- *Obstetrics and Gynecology*
- *Geriatrics*

Specialist Physicians *typically practice in fields such as:*

- *Psychiatry*
- *Surgery*
- *Anesthesiology*
- *Radiology*
- *Cardiology*
- *Oncology*
- *Endocrinology*
- *Hematology*
- *Rheumatology*
- *Neurology*

Sources

Become a PA: Getting Your Prerequisites and Certification. (2019, August 28). Retrieved September 06, 2020, from https://www.aapa.org/career-central/become-a-pa/

Writers, S. (2020, January 21). Physician Assistant Programs & Careers: How to Become a Physician Assistant. Retrieved September 06, 2020, from https://www.learnhowtobecome.org/physician-assistant/

How to Become a Registered Nurse. (2020, September 11). Retrieved September 13, 2020, from https://www.allnursingschools.com/registered-nursing/

Writers, R. (2020, June 15). (APRN) Advanced Practice Registered Nurse - Roles, Programs, Salary Details. Retrieved September 13, 2020, from https://www.registerednursing.org/aprn/

6 Steps to Becoming a Nurse Practitioner: Salary & Programs. (n.d.). Retrieved September 13, 2020, from https://nurse.org/resources/nurse-practitioner/

What is a Medical Assistant? (n.d.). Retrieved September 13, 2020, from https://www.medassistantedu.org/what-is-a-medical-assistant/

What Is a Medical Assistant? (2020, August 07). Retrieved
    September 13, 2020, from
    https://www.allalliedhealthschools.com/medical-
    assisting/what-is-a-medical-assistant/

(n.d.). Retrieved from www.graduate nursingedu.org

Https://www.fsmb.org/siteassets/advocacy/publications/2016c
    ensus.pdf. (n.d.).

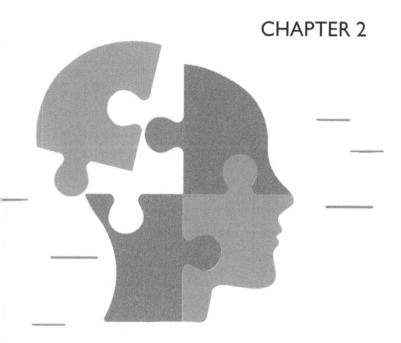

CHAPTER 2

The Initial Visit

2

Completing a new visit with a medical provider can be a daunting experience. New visits, which are known as consultation appointments, typically require more paperwork and time than later visits. While most appointments last 15 to 20 minutes, new patient visits are scheduled for a longer time. Fortunately, there are things that you can do to make sure you get the most out of your visit, and you can use the visit as an opportunity to build a good relationship with your health care provider.

"What should I do before the visit?"

Write down questions for your provider and bring

them to the exam. Bring a list of your medications and doses. Note any unpleasant reactions to medications in the past, even if they are not considered allergic reactions. If you are having a new patient visit with a primary care provider, write down the top three problems that most concern you.

Sometimes there are multiple issues you want to address, either because you developed several symptoms at one time or because of a health care lapse due to loss of insurance. Despite this, there are usually only a few issues that stand out as most important. Write these down and prioritize them. Things that affect your daily activities (such as dizziness or loss of balance), changes in your mental status or thoughts, changes in bodily functions, and worsening pain should go on your priority list. At times, you may not be able to identify which issues are more serious than others. This is okay. If you are unsure, develop a list of symptoms and allow the provider to review them to help determine which items to cover in the initial visit. Issues that can't be covered in the first appointment can be covered in follow-up visits.

The medical visit is a partnership consisting of you and your provider. Taking an active role will empower you in a positive way as you work to achieve and maintain good health.

"I'm meeting a new provider. What can I expect?"

Consolidate your health history prior to the visit. The provider may not need all this information but if they do, you will have it on hand. If you do not, you may find yourself searching through piles of paperwork during the visit, which may take up precious time with the provider. If you do not have your complete health history, attempt to keep copies of your imaging and lab tests. Medical systems are certainly more connected now, but do not assume the new office will have access to your previous records. In some cases, missing health information and studies may prolong or delay treatment.

In compiling your medical history, remember the **Four W's: What, When, Where** and **Why.** You can document the problem you want evaluated by paying attention to these four W's. **What** is the problem? Describe every aspect of the problem. **When** did it start? Along with timing, document the duration of the process. Has it lasted two months, two minutes, or two years? How frequent is the pain or other problem? **Where** is the problem? Describe the area of the body it is located. If you are not able to write down the area, drawing the area can be helpful. Once in the evaluation, you can be more specific by pointing to the area. **Why** has the problem occurred? Were there activities such as exposure to harmful substances or a change in physical activity that may have put you at risk for developing an injury? Falls, eating certain foods, or trauma can cause medical conditions.

When thinking about the 4 W's, ask yourself these questions: How has it affected you? Do you pass out or lose consciousness? The severity of the problem is key to proper evaluation. Does the problem impede your daily activities? Is it a minor blip on your pain scale? Does it affect your mood or ability to understand others? For example, are you depressed from the medical condition or anxious as a result? Did it begin following the initiation of the medication? Have there been any recent changes?

As for the "**when**," a timeline of medical conditions is vital in establishing an accurate and current medical status. Try to create a timeline in chronological order with dates, procedures, and diagnoses. Use medical terms for diagnoses and procedures if possible. Also create a medication list including the dosage, how often you take it, and when you began taking the medication.

Documenting allergies and negative reactions to medications is important. Herbal supplements, vitamins, and over-the-counter pills such as aspirin or ibuprofen are essential information that must be included on your list as they may affect lab work or treatment, or may interact with other medications. If you see a chiropractor, functional medicine doctor, or acupuncturist, this should be relayed to your medical provider. All of this information aides in diagnosis and decision making.

This personal medical history is vital as mentioned, but know your genes, too! This means you should be well versed with your family medical history. It is important to have in-depth knowledge of the medical conditions of your first-degree relatives—your parents, grandparents, aunts and uncles, and brothers and sisters. Both their acute and chronic conditions should be noted.

An acute condition is a medical problem with a rapid onset and short course—for example, appendicitis or pneumonia. A chronic condition is an illness lasting greater than six months that requires ongoing medical attention. Examples of chronic conditions include diabetes, cancer, hypertension, coronary artery disease, and Alzheimer's. Other important information to have is the age your relative was when he or she was diagnosed with the condition and the medications they were placed on. This information may be the missing puzzle piece to your personal diagnosis.

If you have insurance, bring documentation of it. In addition to your primary insurance, you may have Medicaid or Medicare coverage. Most medical offices require this information prior to the visit or on the day of the exam.

Along with having evidence of insurance coverage, it is very helpful for you to know the type of coverage you have and the financial obligations assigned to you by the insurance company. This involves understanding what medical visits the insurance company will cover and what expenses you are responsible for. Health insurers typically reimburse differently for the cost of medical care for an illness versus the cost for an annual exam; and specialty referrals and out-of-network providers are often more expensive than in-network providers. Obtaining this information from your insurance company can lessen your anxiety, your confusion, and ultimately your financial burden.

Know the purpose of the visit. If you are being referred to a specialist, discuss with your primary care doctor the purpose of the referral. If you are referred for a procedure or surgery, know that you may likely have a consultation with the specialist *before* actually scheduling the procedure. There are times when procedures may be done at the initial visit, but if this is the case it is usually specified when the appointment is scheduled.

When able, utilize online patient portal or electronic medical history intake programs prior to your appointment. This will save time and give you more one-on-one time discussing your medical issues with your doctor or nurse.

If you fear that your symptoms or anxiety may interfere with communication between you and the provider, consider asking a trusted family member or friend to go with you to the visit. That individual may be able to assist with the evaluation, and he or she can take notes during the appointment to help you later recall all that the doctor said. Having a family member or friend attend a visit is especially recommended if a patient has memory issues or a cognitive deficit. If someone cannot be physically present with you, video calls may be of use.

"It's time for my appointment. Now what?"

Be on time. Eat prior to the visit unless anticipating blood/lab work. Bring reading material, work, or activities such as cross-word puzzles to pass the time in the waiting room as wait times may vary.

Minimize sensitivity. You will be seen by a health expert whose number one goal is to allow you to have the best medical outcome possible. Providers want you to live a long, fruitful, and healthy life. If recommendations are made that you are sensitive to, evaluate if the suggestions were said or meant maliciously. If they were not, remind yourself that recommendations are meant to get you closer to your health goals and to help you avoid preventable medical problems. Be open to the questions your doctor asks, and receptive to the provider's medical suggestions.

Be honest. It only hinders your health goals to exaggerate, minimize or avoid mentioning details during your doctor's visit. For example, many patients may try to avoid discussing their weight by saying, "Well, I'm just big boned." That may be, but being overweight can be harmful to your health and can place you at risk of developing serious medical conditions.

We are often very sensitive about the life we live, and rightfully so. We have the right to choose the way we live and to enjoy the choices we make. But some of those choices do not promote good health.

The truth is that the way we live is the single most controllable way to prevent certain illnesses and to lessen the need for many medications. Know that if your lifestyle choices are brought up in the visit, it is for your benefit. Be open and perhaps ask yourself why you would not want to change something that is harming your health.

If you have medical issues that you prefer to remain private, talk with your provider about your concern of stigmas and labels associated with certain diagnoses. Along those same lines, it is important to remember that mental health can have a great impact on your general physical health. Good health care includes identifying and treating all health components and that includes our thought patterns and behaviors.

Ask for additional information, if needed. Prior to leaving the visit, especially if you are not clear about things, ask for diagrams, pictorial illustrations, videos or pamphlets to aide your understanding. Please do not feel ashamed if you don't understand certain medical terms or conditions, and never hesitate to ask for information that can help you.

Maintain a professional attitude. There are times when you may know your provider socially, outside of the medical setting. In these cases, it's often best to maintain a division between the social component and the medical evaluation during your visit.

Limit or avoid negative talk about a previous provider. Spending time talking about a previous provider may reduce the time that could otherwise be spent on discussing your current health and on determining a diagnosis and treatment plan. Instead of speaking negatively, address your concerns in a positive way. For example, if you felt like you were rushed with previous doctor visits, comment to your new provider about your concern for having adequate time with them.

"I don't want to have to tell my story again."

No one wants to keep telling the same story over

and over again, and compiling your complete medical history can be time-consuming. But the beauty of having done your medical history homework is that now you have it, and you only need to update it as your situations evolves.

You'll also find that having two different versions—a short, abbreviated version and an extended version—can prevent you from feeling that you have to repeat the story over and over again. The short version can be used for intake, and the longer version can guide the discussion with your provider. You may want to tell the provider every detail surrounding an occurrence, but this can take up valuable time. Let your detailed medical history do much of the work, and when talking to your provider try to remain focused on your symptoms or on answering your provider's specific questions.

Now that the visit has concluded, consider these questions when determining if you will continue to partner with them in the future: Do you trust your doctor? How does he or she put you at ease? Is it because of the same ethnicity, gender, socioeconomic status, or is it through an ease of communication?

Sometimes, you can have a less than desirable experience with a health care provider. Always be an advocate for yourself. If you were mistreated, discuss your concerns with the appropriate entity or manager.

Remember, taking all of the things mentioned in this chapter into account will set you up for a productive and informative initial visit. Hopefully, you can establish a good rapport with your provider. This can be helpful in building a foundation of faith in them and in your partnership.

Key Points

- Get off to a good start by being prepared with a complete medical history and taking it to your appointment.

- Write down questions and symptoms prior to your visit.

- Be honest and descriptive with your symptoms and concerns.

- Remain open and receptive to your provider's suggestions during your visit.

- Ask for additional resources (informational brochures, etc.), if needed.

Surgeries
and Procedures

3

Some medical conditions require surgical intervention. An invasive procedure or surgery can be a scary, anxiety-provoking thought. You may have had a previous bad experience in surgery, or you may fear undergoing anesthesia. You may also wonder if you'll feel any pain during the procedure, or even if you will not wake up. But the vast majority of surgeries go exceptionally well, and in most cases they are necessary in order for a patient to regain good health. However, some surgeries are done that are not medically required and are thus considered elective. Cosmetic surgeries are an example of this and are usually not covered by insurance.

"I need surgery. Now what?"

Having questions and concerns about surgery is normal. In fact, you should always ask questions: *"Is this surgery required? Will it be life-saving? What will happen if I don't have it?"*

Before any surgery or procedure, you should establish how necessary the procedure is. When your doctor recommends a surgery or procedure, discuss how it will treat the condition. Explore alternatives. Inquire about the success versus failure rate. Additional questions you may want answers to include:

- Will the procedure completely take care of my medical condition or simply improve it?
- What is the medical name for the procedure, and what does the procedure entail?
- Are there videos or simulations of the procedure that would help me better understand what to expect? (Companies that make a

device/instrument used in a procedure often produce videos describing its use.)

- What kind of anesthesia will I have, if any?
- Will the procedure be done in the office, in the hospital, or in a surgery center? Should I check my insurance to determine if it prefers one setting versus the other for the surgery?
- What's the average time duration for the surgery? Is an overnight stay at the hospital required?
- What are the potential complications and how frequent do these complications occur?
- Are there options other than this surgical procedure that would accomplish the same cure? What options are the least invasive, with the fewest complications?
- What is the recovery time? What can I expect immediately following the procedure?
- Will pain medication or antibiotics be given following the procedure?
- When should I return for a follow-up?

- After the surgery, how soon can I expect my condition to improve? Will I experience immediate relief?
- Will I need a caregiver following my surgery?
- When can I return to routine activity, i.e., work, exercise, sex?
- What if I reconsider and decide not to have the procedure? Is there a charge if I change my mind and cancel the procedure?

Before you make the final decision to have a surgery or procedure, you should also consider how it may affect your other health conditions. For major surgeries, it is recommended to have clearance from your primary care doctor and/or certain specialists. A couple of reasons are if you have a high-risk condition such as heart disease or take medications that impact bleeding during a surgery. For instance, blood thinners may need to be discontinued for a specific period of time prior to the surgery to avoid complications. Some conditions—such as smoking, diabetes and obesity—may increase the risk of infection, increase the chance of anesthesia complications, or affect the healing rate.

If you anticipate having surgery, consider improving your health as much as you can. Get proper rest, optimize your nutrition and water intake, decrease stress, and strategize to improve your mood. Recent research studies identify a patient's mood on entering a surgical procedure as an important factor in determining if the patient develops chronic post-surgical pain. A certain level of concern about a surgery is normal and expected. But for patients with elevated anxiety, negative thought patterns, and depression, healing rates are slowed and development of chronic pain is more likely. Repeating positive affirmations and implementing other coping strategies for stress may help prevent negative outcomes.

Scheduling a pre-operative visit is important. This is the time to ask last minute questions. A family member should be present to hear the details. A review of current and past medical problems and medications is vital at this visit as well, so that your surgeon will be as prepared as possible for any situation that may arise when you are under anesthesia. (The medical history you created, as discussed in Chapter 2, will be helpful here.)

At your pre-op visit, the medical office should provide pre-surgery instructions especially for the night prior to and the day of the procedure. It is also a good idea to schedule a post-procedure follow-up appointment now.

You can prepare for the post-procedure period by developing strategies for a smooth as possible recovery. This can entail enlisting assistance from family or friends to check on you or to help you with aftercare, to modifying your home to make it easier for you to achieve daily needs (dressing, bathing, and eating). Go through your home to identify and eliminate potential fall risks (get rid of loose rugs, set up a shower chair, etc.). Consider your meals post-procedure. Some surgeries may call for diet restrictions after the operation, so inquire about any dietary instructions ahead of time. But in general, you can optimize good nutrition with easily absorbed foods such as soups, many of which can be made on a large scale with minimal effort. Hydration post-procedure is important and all too easily overlooked.

Note that if you develop any new medical issues or experience a change to an existing medical condition after your pre-operative appointment but prior to your procedure, it is vital to inform your surgeon. Bladder infections, respiratory infections, a fever, or bleeding changes should be reported right away.

"The procedure is over. Now what!?"

Many people assume the highest risks are during the procedure. But the post-procedure time can hold just as much risk. The first days and hours after a surgery pose the highest chance of complications. Keep your discharge instructions close by so you can routinely refer to them, and be diligent in following them. Closely monitor for changes in your health status outside the anticipated effects. Examine the surgical site daily for signs of infection, and be on the watch for an elevated body temperature or a change in your mental status. Anything out of the ordinary, including pain outside the normal severity or expected length of time, should warrant a discussion with your provider.

Limitations after surgery are typically reviewed by the doctor who performed the surgery, or by his or her nurse or PA. Sometimes stairs should be avoided, and other times submersion in water should be avoided for a certain period of time to allow surgical wounds to heal. Showers are often recommended over baths, but other methods to clean your body should be discussed with your provider. Some patients will need to monitor water temperature. Hot showers are not recommended for patients following heart procedures since hot water can cause the blood vessels to dilate, making blood pressure drop and resulting in dizziness and feeling faint.

Prepare for some degree of pain following a surgery. The goal of pain medication is to decrease and control the pain but not necessarily to take the pain away 100%. Remember this when taking pain medications, especially narcotics which may be habit-forming. Other types of pain medications are frequently used in their place or to supplement smaller doses of narcotics to control the pain post-procedure.

Activity level is a key component of recovery from a surgery. Too much activity too fast can disrupt sutures, hinder wound healing, and cause other setbacks. On the other hand, too little movement can increase your risk of developing blood clots in the legs or lungs. Blood clots are a severe, life-threatening complication which should be taken seriously. Post-surgical activity level is something that was likely discussed prior to your operation, but if you have questions about what's appropriate and what is not, do not hesitate to ask. You want to know what activities are recommended to promote recovery, and by the same token you want to be aware of movements to avoid. Expect to feel weak after a lengthy procedure or hospital admission. Know that it may take some time to get stronger, and rather than focusing on what you can't do, focus on what you *can* do.

Realize that breathing is often impacted by surgeries. Anesthesia or simply changes due to pain and positioning can affect how deeply you breathe. Moreover, when in pain, most people tend to take shallow breaths which causes a decrease in oxygen flow to body tissues. Shallow breathing also limits lung expansion and can lead to complications such as pneumonia.

Sometimes, you can do everything right and still have complications. If complications arise, contact the doctor immediately. The healing process can be easy for some and very difficult for others. Avoid comparing yourself to others. Each person heals differently. You have your own course, so never get discouraged. The goal is to heal completely and to gain optimal health.

Key Points

- Know procedure details: options, risks, preparation, and recovery times.

- Tell your doctor about any health changes prior to the surgery.

- Follow post-procedural instructions to facilitate faster healing and minimize complications.

- Recovery may be more challenging than the procedure itself.

Time for a
New Doctor

4

Each individual—whether they are a patient or a medical provider—is unique and has their own distinct personality. Personalities play an integral role in the development of all relationships, and the patient–doctor relationship is no different. Healthcare is a personal journey and is a sensitive matter. And is important for you to feel comfortable with your provider. But sometimes your personalities simply do not mesh.

Often times, there are particular attributes a patient is looking for in a provider. For example, a physician's bedside manner may or may not be important to you. The empathetic, hand-holding provider may not be your cup of tea, while a no-

nonsense person may be more your speed. These preferences are real and valid. Don't do yourself a disservice by feeling shame or guilt for wanting to feel confident and at ease with your provider. Choose one who suits you the best.

A provider's goal should always be to help a patient achieve optimal health. When evaluating whether your doctor is a good fit, consider these questions:

- Does your provider listen and communicate effectively?
- Are you comfortable enough in the provider's presence to divulge your entire medical history, or are you fearful to speak up when discussing symptoms?
- Are chronic illnesses and allergic reactions considered when medications are prescribed or changed?
- Does your provider display personal bias, either economic, ethical, racial or religious?

- Are you confident in the provider's knowledge, skill, and decision making?
- Can you get in touch with your provider when you need to?

If the comfort level you want is not there or the fit does not seem right, what is the best route to take? This can be a delicate situation, and searching for a new doctor can be fraught with anxiety. So before switching providers, consider addressing your concerns with your current doctor. The concerns may stem from simple communication problems that can easily be resolved.

Sometimes, it is the provider's office staff that is problematic. If you are unhappy about office logistics such as a lack of friendliness or a lack of timely response to your phone calls, you may want to talk to your provider or his or her office manager. Some office protocols and policies may be outside the practitioner's control (due to insurance or legal requirements), but many office protocols can be modified.

You may call and say, "I want to speak personally to my doctor," but remember that providers are usually with other patients during the day until 5 PM or even later. Because of this, most exchange of information is done at the end of the day. Or you may wonder why your doctor's medical assistant, rather than your doctor, calls with test results. Avoid dwelling on *who* gives the information as long as the information is timely and given in a comprehensive manner.

It is sometimes unrealistic to expect rapid turnaround time for call-backs or emails. Discuss with your provider average call back times and other policies that may affect your care. Sharing expectations with your existing doctor may prevent you from needless discontent. If you choose another provider, consider discussing this during the initial evaluation.

"When is it time to change providers?"

When you've addressed your concerns with the

provider and are still disheartened, or when you are no longer comfortable with him or her, it may be a good idea to look for someone new. This will be evident when you all are no longer working as a team. Healthcare maintenance and treatment require a cohesive team approach by you and your provider, whether that is a doctor, nurse practitioner or physician assistant. And sometimes your needs change with time. Initially, a family medicine practitioner may have covered your health maintenance. But as you age and develop new medical conditions, it may be more beneficial for you to have a specialist as your primary provider.

When the decision has been made to transition to another provider, seek word-of-mouth recommendations from people that you know and/or ask your insurance company for preferred providers. Once you find the right fit, notify your existing provider's office. A records release from their care is required for the new provider to obtain your medical chart. Most hospitals and surgery centers require a release of information prior to sending these documents as well. Providing the most accurate and up-to-date medical history will ensure you get off on the right foot with the new provider of choice.

"When should I get a second opinion?"

Unfortunately, some medical conditions and circumstances are not straightforward. Treatment options vary and are not always simple to understand. Another medical provider may offer different approaches and methods to treat a problem. This is when a second opinion comes into play.

A second opinion can serve many purposes and provide you with additional information and perspective. Your goal is to obtain clear and concise knowledge about your medical condition, treatment plan, and potential progression.

Only you—the patient—can determine if you feel well informed or not, and if you have confidence in the person caring for you. Regardless, patients commonly hesitate before asking their doctor about getting a second opinion. People often wonder, *"Is it wrong to want a second opinion? Does it imply I don't trust my doctor? Will I be penalized for this? Will my doctor think that I'm worried about his or her being old or not up to speed? Will my provider think I'm just looking for someone to agree with me?"*

Generally, medical providers are understanding of the request. All physicians take an oath to provide the best medical care and to do no harm. Providing excellent patient care is most doctors' primary concern. And if a medical provider is confident in his or her assessment, he/she will welcome a second opinion to affirm their diagnosis, treatment plan or recommended medication. A provider's ego should never be a factor—if it is, it may be a problem.

Often times, a patient will be reassured that the initial medical provider did everything and ran every appropriate test. But remember, no two providers are equal in breath of knowledge, experience, or surgical skills. As a patient, you should want confirmation that all options have been explored and exhausted. The ball is in your court. You have a voice.

Key Points

- Attempt to develop a solid, professional relationship with your provider.

- Look for a medical provider whom you're comfortable with and who meets your needs.

- A provider's office management and staff can influence satisfaction with your doctor; don't neglect to address any concerns regarding these issues.

- Second opinions are a valuable resource and option.

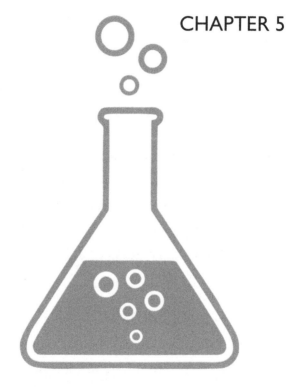

CHAPTER 5

Medications

5

Most patients want a cure for their medical condition. However, today many patients tend to want a more "natural" remedy and believe that all medications can cause additional problems or are generally bad for you. Thus, medications and patients have a love-hate relationship.

It is certainly correct that all medicines have the potential to cause side effects. And because every person is genetically different, the same medicine may affect one person differently than someone else. It is important to know your body and its response to common medications.

"Are these medications safe?"

Medications can interact with other medicines, or with even herbal supplements. The brain-preserving fish oil supplement or the senna tea you take for constipation may have additional effects that you do not even realize. If you consume daily anti-inflammatory medicines like ibuprofen, it can affect the body's response to prescribed medicines or even to treatments and procedures. Carefully research your herbal supplements, over-the-counter medications, and your medical conditions to ensure that taking the supplements will not be harmful. Pharmacists can provide you with a list of medications to avoid while completing the prescription. Review this information prior to taking the prescription.

Remember that your local pharmacist can be a helpful, supplemental resource for information about your medications. However, a pharmacist is not a medical provider. His or her role is to inform you of vital information regarding the prescription that your doctor ordered. Questions about your particular condition in relationship to the prescribed medication should go to the doctor who wrote it.

Also be advised that an internet search can provide research articles and other educational tools for patients. However, this information should be used only to supplement the advice of your doctor. Your doctors have studied and obtained advanced degrees, completed years of training, and likely many years of clinical experience in the medical field. They are the experts.

It's important to talk to your doctor about your prescription, because the same medication can be used to treat several different conditions and diseases. Take, for example, Topamax. Topamax can be prescribed to treat migraines, nerve pain or for weight loss. These are all very different medical conditions that can be treated with the same medication. Your pharmacist is most likely not aware of what specific medical condition you are experiencing.

It is best to discuss your concerns about any medications with your doctor when he or she first prescribes them. If you develop hesitancies about the medication later, call your provider to discuss those fears. Serious complications can occur when certain medications are suddenly stopped, so ask about those when you are first prescribed a medication and consult your provider before stopping it. Ultimately you may end up discussing these issues with select office staff if the provider is not available.

It is natural to be skeptical about medications or treatments. This is especially true if you know someone who has had a negative experience. Use this information and discuss the concerns with the provider so you can make the best decision.

Now that you are comfortable with the medication, develop an easy system to remember to take it. Incorporate it into your previously established daily routine. This limits the stress of potentially missing a dose of medication.

Some medications are intended to be continued for long periods of time. Other medications are prescribed for a short period of time. For all medications, it is very important to complete the course as directed unless side effects or allergic reactions occur. The desired health benefit—such as getting rid of an infection—is directly related to completion of the medication. You may a think finishing an antibiotic prescription is not necessary if your pain or redness is gone, but that would be a mistake.

"I'm having side effects. Now what should I do?"

Each person responds to medications differently. And often side effects are the first indication of when to discontinue a medicine. For some, reading the long list of a medicine's potential side effects can provoke anxiety. However, it is important to recognize if they occur. Common side effects are nausea, vomiting, changes in sleep pattern and rashes. Be aware of mood changes, escalation of pain, or severe fatigue. More severe and potentially life threatening side effects may include shortness of breath and swelling of the face or lips. Contact your medical provider immediately with development of side effects. Some side effects are minor, but mention them nonetheless.

Most side effects will occur early on after starting a medication. But some-like muscle cramps with cholesterol lowering medications—may develop weeks or months later. Review common short term vs. long term side effects.

Yearly visits with your primary care provider or specialist are a good time to reevaluate the need for medications. Depression, hypertension, and migraines are just a few examples of conditions that can change over the course of a year or two. Lifestyle changes, eliminating life stressors, or weight loss may contribute to decreasing or discontinuing a medication.

It is helpful to keep a list of medications and the conditions they are treating. Update this when any changes occur. Though we are in an electronic age, it is advantageous to keep a printed list on hand. Family members or a support person may need to provide the medication list in the event you become ill.

Finally, safeguard your medications. Many medications have the potential for abuse, or they can be life-threatening in the case of an accidental overdose. This is particularly true of sedatives, pain medications, and blood pressure medications.

Key Points

- Know the condition the medication is treating.

- Know the most common side effects of the medication.

- Discuss any fear of taking the medication with your doctor during your office visit, and if concerns later arise at home, contact the office.

- Keep a hard copy of your medications for quick reference and so that others can assist if needed.

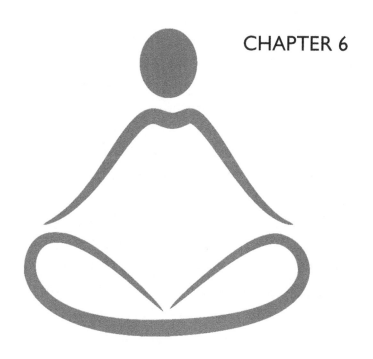

CHAPTER 6

Managing Expectations

6

"I came to be fixed. Why can't you fix me?"

Frustrating, isn't it? We live in a very convenient world where there's an easy fix for almost anything. The screen on your smartphone cracks? Just drop it by a repair shop or mail it in, and get a new screen. So in a world where so many things can be fixed or replaced, it is no wonder we get frustrated by limitations regarding the human body. We are living, breathing complex beings. When something goes wrong with the body, surgery can sometimes provide the answer as a "quick fix", but not always. After all, we are not machines.

Often times, the expectation for a medical visit is to leave the appointment with a diagnosis and a treatment plan that will completely resolve the problem. However, many times diagnosis requires not only a clinical exam but also blood tests, and sometimes x-rays or more complex radiologic studies. Commonly, the battery of tests needed for a full diagnosis is not done on the same day as the first discussion of the problem with your provider. Tests may require preparation on the patient's part and involve other doctors. While simple imaging studies typically don't require much patient preparation, other tests can be more involved. Fasting or drinking a preparatory medication may be mandatory for tests such as a colonoscopy or a barium enema swallow.

After completing a diagnostic test, the amount of time it takes to get the results can vary widely. Blood test results can take several days to several weeks. Imaging tests generally take longer since a radiologist must read the image and then send the report to the patient's doctor. The doctor then has to review the report, which can add several more days to the time before the patient finally receives the results.

Rarely are results instantaneous or immediate, and little can be done to speed the process. Being mentally prepared for the wait, and not allowing yourself to become too anxious, can help. Once all the test results are in, you are one step closer to a diagnosis.

It also helps to be patient regarding return phone calls and responses to emails. Each provider's office has a different way of operating and different response times. Familiarize yourself with expected call back times to avoid miscommunication and frustration. Since most doctors and other providers are seeing patients or are in surgery all day, their ability to get back in touch with you quickly, and on the same day you call, may be limited. Many times patient phone calls will be returned at the end of the day by nurses or other office staff. Emergent situations and conditions always take precedence, and a medical provider will almost always notify you quickly if he or she thinks your condition is alarming and requires urgent attention.

Overall, the goal is to get a swift and clear diagnosis. But it sometimes takes weeks or months to determine exactly what is wrong and develop a treatment plan. Even then, there are times when your provider cannot determine a diagnosis, despite his or her best efforts. In those cases, referral to a specialist for further testing is often the next step. With an unknown diagnosis, consider performing your own research and/or seeking an evaluation at an academic medical center. Don't underestimate your capacity to participate in your healthcare.

"Do I need a follow-up appointment?"

Follow-up appointments may be scheduled to discuss your test results and diagnosis and to relay any important information. The follow-up appointment is a good time to ask additional questions. Questions regarding treatment should focus on medications, procedures, or alternative management options. For example, ask about the anticipated time to cure the infection, stop the bleeding, or make a rash go away. Is the disease or treatment dependent on diet or activity level? Are there physical limitations while the treatment is in progress?

You will also want to know if the condition is acute (i.e., temporary) or chronic (i.e., something which cannot be cured and is long term). With conditions that are chronic, healthcare goals usually shift to preventing or lessening symptoms from the illness, so as to create a better quality of life.

If the treatment plan involves surgery, realize that outcomes may vary. Surgery is traumatic to the body and unwanted changes can occur. For example, scar tissue and chronic pain can develop after surgery. This sometimes cannot be predicted. It is important to discuss the benefits of surgery and the anticipated healing time. Although there are risks involved, in many cases, surgery may be your best option.

The treatment course may vary from person to person despite the same diagnosis. No two people are alike. Discuss your provider's treatment goals and determine if they are consistent with your goals. If you do not have goals for your treatment, take time to establish some. Remain focused on the goals you have set. Often a good approach is to gauge your progress by comparing today versus a month or a year ago.

At the follow-up appointment, discuss any frustrations or concerns regarding your diagnosis with the provider. Prolonged feelings of frustration and anxiety can manifest in the body and cause other health problems, potentially worsening the illness you are seeking treatment for.

Before you leave the visit, ask yourself if you

engaged in meaningful dialogue with your provider and have had all your questions answered. Are you leaving the office with a sense of accomplishment? Ultimately, your goal is to leave the visit knowing the next steps in your care, whether that includes more testing, a new medication, a procedure, or a referral to a specialist.

Key Points

- Manage your expectations. Realize that establishing a correct diagnosis may take time.

- Results from lab work or imaging may not be immediately available.

- Office protocols may limit direct access to the provider outside of an office visit.

- After the diagnosis, you and your provider can work together to develop a treatment plan.

CHAPTER 7

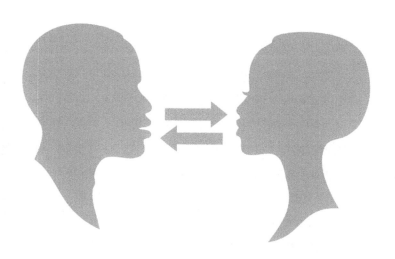

Communicating
Effectively

7

Have you ever left a doctor's office and felt like you didn't know what the take-home points were? Well, you are not alone. It happens more than you think. It can be a lot of information to absorb at once. Problems can occur if you leave without all the information or with a misunderstanding. The confusion can come from the sheer amount of information provided, how it was presented, or from the words themselves.

"Are we speaking the same language?"

The type of words we hear can easily be a barrier in communication. Medical jargon can sound like a different language. If your provider uses a lot of medical terms, do not be shy or fearful to let them know you don't understand. Ask if they can paraphrase it in layman terms so that you can fully understand. However, it's a good idea to write down the medical term or diagnosis for future research and discussion. Sometimes, providers assume patients understand medical terms when they don't, so don't be afraid to speak up and ask!

Misinterpretation can occur by both parties in a medical office visit. Confirming the provider has a clear understanding about the issues you are concerned about is key. A patient's history and symptoms may be reviewed multiple times during a visit to prevent mistakes. This can be frustrating, since it seems repetitious, but it's worth the effort to make sure everything is recorded correctly. It's easy to misinterpret information, and a recap—or visit summary— can ensure the information is correct. The keys points in a visit summary should include presumed diagnosis, planned tests, and anticipated treatment. Some offices provide a written summary for each patient.

There are several ways to communicate in a productive way. These can include using nonverbal signs such as good body language and eye contact. Avoiding distractions such as cell phones during an office visit can show you are fully invested. Though, you should not have to prove to the provider that you have real issues with your health.

Communication is often compromised when too much emotion is involved. If you go into an office visit assuming your doctor thinks you are you dishonest, productive dialogue may be limited. It's always best to enter the visit with confidence that your symptoms will be addressed seriously.

Deep sadness about a diagnosis or anger from unmet expectations are common, but it may be difficult to communicate when these emotions surface. Try to avoid coming to your visit angry. If these feelings arise and hinder communication, your provider may decide to discontinue the visit. Raising your voice, using profanity, or threatening the provider will end any productive dialogue and may lead to your removal from the office. Anger prevents active listening. Threats—whether violent or nonviolent—derail a provider's focus from solving your health concerns to protection of self, staff and the office.

During your office visit, speak for yourself if at all possible. Family members and spouses are there for support and to provide supplemental information regarding your care. For example, family members may see changes in your behavior that you do not notice. But overall, the provider wants to hear from you, in your own words, as much as possible.

If you are physically unable to speak, patient advocates are invaluable. Likewise, if you and your doctor speak different languages, a translator will be required. Although ideally you and your medical provider will speak the same language, that is not always the case. Notify the office before your visit to have a non-family member interpreter present if English is your second language. You may know English well, but when treatment is discussed, details can be missed or misinterpreted. Be aware. Family members may paraphrase, rather than translate directly, which may influence the message you hear or what the provider is told.

Intake forms filled out prior to talking to your provider are important nonverbal tools used to communicate concerns. When completing the forms, be specific and give as much detail as possible. Avoid minimizing symptoms and their impact on you.

Dishonest reports or discussions about dietary intake and elevated blood sugars, especially for patients with conditions like diabetes, are detrimental. Acknowledging non-compliance with medications can steer your medical provider to the best treatment or alternatives. It is possible that you may be better suited for a weekly or monthly medication, rather than a daily medication. Your honesty will optimize compliance and how well the medicine works. Iron infusions are a good example of this. Daily iron supplements can cause constipation and therefore decrease compliance, whereas iron infusions every 6-8 weeks may be a better option for the treatment of iron-deficiency anemia.

Communicating mental health changes whether limited to mood changes or more substantial mental deterioration must be relayed to the provider. Specific symptoms and details are needed. Likewise, your sexual history may be daunting to discuss, but divulging a complete history can make a difference. Honesty regarding lifestyles can aide in proper diagnosis, effective treatment, and an understanding of your risk factors. Many patients are concerned about sexually transmitted infections (STIs), but other diseases can also result from certain lifestyles.

"I feel like I'm not being heard."

Every book about effective communication encourages active listening. This type of involved listening is imperative for physicians and patients alike. Listen with the intent to learn. For example, a provider may discuss an issue with one intent, but you may interpret it completely different. A doctor may say you are overweight and recommend dietary changes, but you may interpret this as being told you are fat and lazy. Such assumptions can be a major barrier in effectively receiving information beneficial to your health. A receptive attitude will give additional insight to your condition and will improve communication with your provider.

Key Points

- If you are asked to review your medical history or medications more than once, be patient and understanding.

- If English is your second language, ask for formal language assistance (a translator) prior to your office visit.

- Nonverbal communication, such as positive body language and putting away your cell phone, can have a beneficial impact on your visit.

- Be willing to provide sensitive medical history to assist with proper diagnosis and treatment.

- A visit summary may avoid miscommunication and misinformation.

CHAPTER 8

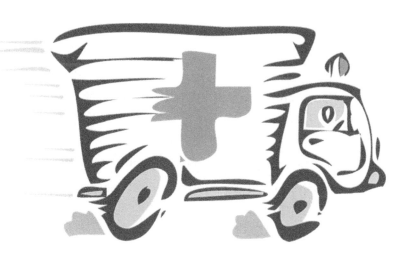

Emergency
Room Visits

8

"Does going to the ER have to be such an ordeal?"

Life is unpredictable. Motor vehicle accidents, chest pain, loss of consciousness and traumas occur unexpectedly. Often, harrowing or painful events like these leave you wondering what to do.

When you are not feeling well, it may be necessary to go the emergency room. But sometimes it is hard to know whether you should rush to the ER, or whether you can wait to see your regular doctor.

It helps to remember that the emergency room is designed to treat and manage emergent medical conditions. In this case, emergent refers to conditions that are potentially life-threatening or can cause permanent damage if they are not treated right away. Emergency room visits are not for health care maintenance.

Going to an emergency room when it's not necessary can actually be counterproductive. On the other hand, if you feel you or a loved one needs to go to the ER, don't let dread of the unknown, fear of looking foolish, or a desire to avoid a potentially long wait time keep you away. Never delay or avoid seeking immediate medical attention when necessary.

Once you get to the emergency room, know that the ER visit is a different kind of beast from a routine office visit. Stakes are higher and emotions are at a peak. When you or someone you care for is actively deteriorating, you simply want the fastest and best treatment.

Emergency room providers will have one goal: to

stabilize the emergent condition. Sometimes, a concrete diagnosis can be made. Other times, an ER evaluation will only identify the active, acute problem and to prevent it from getting worse. Often the emergency lies in the symptoms of a poorly controlled condition such as diabetes or hypertension. The ER providers will seek to alleviate those symptoms to avoid even more severe complications.

A good way to navigate an emergency room visit is to first stay calm. Try to focus on the developing medical situation. This is important whether you are the one in need or you are the person escorting a family member or friend. A calm demeanor will allow you to communicate effectively. You will want to clearly explain the events leading to the situation, how the condition developed, and the patient's medical history. A lack of accurate or complete information can delay treatment.

In addition to articulating the current medical problem, it's also important to tell the ER providers the medications you take and their dosage. Also provide the name of the doctor who typically manages your medical issue, because the emergency medicine providers may want to consult him or her regarding aid for your care. Having the doctor's contact information can save time. Above all, remember that accurate details and honest communication of events leading to the emergency will speed the process of getting the necessary help.

If you are a patient, it is helpful to have someone with you to provide support and to be an advocate on your behalf. It can be a friend, family member, or even co-worker who assists you in time of need. Your companion may transport you to the ER so that you don't have to drive, can serve as an interpreter, or can assist by contacting family members. Most people are willing to help a friend or colleague. Utilize them as needed. And, of course, utilize the ER when appropriate.

Key Points

- Emergency room visits are for emergency care, not for routine health care or non-urgent medical conditions.

- Remain as calm as possible during emergency evaluations.

- Take a list of your medications.

- Bring a support person to help you during the ER visit.

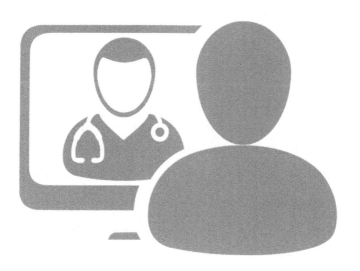

CHAPTER 9

Telemedicine

9

Life has changed. Due to the Covid-19 pandemic, telemedicine has garnered a great deal of interest over a relatively short period of time. Virtual visits via computer or smartphone are being used more and more for a number of reasons.They limit the physical person-to-person contact between patients and staff, thus reducing the possibility of spreading infection.

Even though in-person visits may be restricted, the need for health maintenance has not diminished. Many medical offices have created new protocols to help you maintain your health, and may offer virtual visits as an option. If that's the case, preparation for a telemedicine meeting is beneficial.

"How will virtual visits help me?"

Telemedicine is a tool for evaluation without entering the doctor's office, and a virtual visit gives you access to your medical provider without any risk. Physical examinations cannot be done or are limited during a virtual visit, however your provider may still be able to make diagnoses based on your conversation. Lab test results and imaging results can be discussed in detail during a virtual visit. Counseling for many conditions and medication education can be easily completed using telemedicine as well.

There are several ways to maximize your virtual medical visit:

1. Remember that telemedicine visits are equivalent in importance to an in-office visit. The visits can result in a diagnosis of a new problem, and/or the development of a

plan of care.

2. Prepare for virtual visits as you would for an in-office visit by having your medical history at hand, and making a list of questions you want to discuss with your provider.

3. Find a quiet space in your home that allows you to communicate without distractions. If you are outside the home, try to find a private location for a discussion of potentially sensitive topics.

4. Establish a secure internet connect and an environment with good lighting.

5. Review connection instructions prior to the scheduled appointment time.

6. Prepare to answer calls at or around the appointment time, anticipating it is the doctor's office. Be aware that the telemedicine call may be marked as originating from an unknown or restricted phone number.

7. Wear clothing that will allow for appropriate potential visualization of your problem area.

8. Have ready any medical equipment potentially needed during a visit: a blood pressure
   cuff, glucometer, thermometer, scale, etc.

Virtual visits may be here to stay. Do your best to
get the most out of them.

Key Points

- Virtual office visits with your medical provider
  are just as important as in-person visits.

- Ensure your phone or computer is working and
  ready for the call.

- Prepare as you would for any in-office visit by
  having your medical history, list of medications,
  and a list of questions at hand.

CHAPTER 10

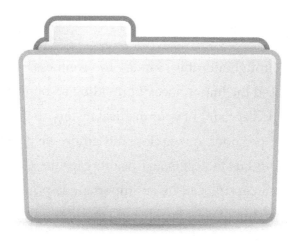

Creating a
Health Capsule

10

Throughout this guide to wellness, we've stressed the importance of providing an honest and detailed account of your medical history to the doctor or provider. As we close this guide, we'll look at how to create a personal health capsule. Creating such a capsule can be an important step in taking ownership of your health and your life.

"Why should I do this? I can remember everything that has happened!"

We all too often assume we will be able to recall our medical history perfectly, in great detail, whenever needed, and on a moment's notice. Unfortunately, this is rarely the case. Have you ever had to rummage through paperwork to find a doctor's name? Or been flustered when asked to name the medications you take, and their dosage? Many times, we link a diagnosis to another life event or important date in our lives. For example, you may remember the year your diabetes was diagnosed because it was a few days before your cousin's wedding or right before an anniversary trip you had planned. Medical memories can be prompted in this fashion—but an office visit is not the right time to 'go down memory lane!' When having an appointment with your doctor, time is limited and must be used wisely.

"So, what's a health capsule?"

A health capsule includes a concise timeline and explanation of medical diagnoses, surgeries, hospitalizations, and medications. A timeline not only illustrates the medical problems in one's life but can highlight a disease's progression. And if your doctor is well versed with your history, it will be easier for him or her to manage your current medical issues.

The timeline should include a list of all prior diagnoses. It should also include a complete list of medications that you have taken in the past, when they were started and stopped, and your reactions to them. If you have had an allergic reaction or unpleasant side effects to a medication, this should be included in the health capsule. Likewise, if a medication improved your condition, that information should be recorded as well. Such information will prevent you being prescribed similar medications that could either be dangerous or not useful.

Timelines are particularly valuable in treating chronic conditions, such as lung disease or diabetes. Peaks flows in lung disease track lung function, whereas hemoglobin A1c monitors control of blood sugars in diabetes. Timelines of these functions can give your provider a better overall view of your health history and how current symptoms factor in.

Begin creating your health capsule by keeping all documents related to your medical care. In addition to keeping all operative reports from major surgeries such as cardiac stent placement and bypass surgeries, keep records from procedures such as endoscopies, colonoscopies, bladder studies, EEGs, EKGs, and nerve studies. Also keep reports from imaging studies such as X-rays, ultrasounds, MRIs, CT scans, and mammograms. Save copies of all your blood tests. Lab values are important because they can help monitor your medical conditions and provide insight.

"Where can I get all this information?"

If you haven't done so in the past, now is the time to get in the habit of keeping all records from your doctor or hospital visits. For past medical records that you have not kept, contact your medical provider's office. Most offices are willing to provide your medical documents, but often you must take the initiative to ask.

To make things easier, many medical offices now

have computer applications through which patients can access their medical records. These programs allow patients to log into a portal or database to view lab and diagnostic test results, visit summaries, and previous and future appointments. Even if this information is available online, it's a good idea to keep a printed copy in your files as part of your health capsule. You can also use your full health care capsule to create a short, condensed version that you carry in your wallet in case of emergency. The condensed version should have a list of your serious medical conditions or allergies and a list of your medications.

The information may seem overwhelming and full of unfamiliar jargon. But the goal is to have access, be informed, and actively participate in your health care journey. The capsule you have created will also be a valuable resource for your medical provider. Take the portfolio or collection with you to an initial visit, realizing that the provider is unlikely to sit and review it immediately but nonetheless is important to have.

Key Points

In creating your health capsule:

- Create categories by medical condition. For each condition, keep a chronological record of the month and year of diagnosis, lab test results, the medications prescribed for it, any procedures undertaken, and your symptoms.

- List each surgical procedure with its date, including the month and the year.

- Place diagnoses, procedures, and tests in chronological order.

- Update the capsule periodically, adding documents when available.

- Keep your medical documents in one place where they can easily be located.

AFTERWORD

"What comes next for my health care?"

We hope this guide will motivate you to take charge of your health and initiate positive steps towards well-being. Keep your goals in mind. Better health translates to improved energy, improved mood, and more focus. It allows freedom to enjoy the things you love in life. Ask your doctor which areas of your health are of most concern. The more you know, the better equipped you are to make sound decisions between medical visits.

Take an active role in learning about your health. If you do not understand something about a diagnosis, talk to your provider. You can ask the provider for information about a particular condition, and also take steps to learn about the diagnosis or disease on your own. If you seek out information on the internet, make sure you visit reputable medical sites. Although much information on the Internet is good, some is tainted with inaccuracies and generalizations. Be strategic with your information sources, and confirm the accuracy of the information you find.

Avoid being overly critical or anxious about every detail of your health. This can be just as detrimental as not paying any attention to your well-being. Unfounded worry can lead to unnecessary tests, procedures, and surgeries which cause undue risk. Anxiety and stress can also manifest in physical abnormalities and can exacerbate some conditions. Speak with your health provider about your concerns, so that he or she can guide you towards appropriate monitoring of your condition. Just as weighing yourself daily is not recommended or productive during a weight loss journey, over-involvement with every detail of your health may be counterproductive. The degree of involvement will be different for everyone.

If you have an on-going medical condition, consider joining a support group to learn more about your condition and how other people manage it. Make use of all opportunities to educate, empower and encourage yourself.

Regardless of your current health level, always be intentional in your dietary decisions and exercise levels. Remember to keep track of medical records, and always prepare ahead to make the most out of all your medical visits—whether in-person or virtual. Your health is important. It is invaluable and deserves dedicated attention.

Don't rob yourself of the opportunity to take your health by the reins.

ACKNOWLEDGMENTS

We thank God whom placed it in our hearts to write this guide. May He continue to utilize our gifts in order to give Him the glory.

There are countless people whom have encouraged and inspired us in this endeavor. We would like to thank Cara Frye, Danyel Hagens MD, Taura Long MD, Beverly Moore, Paris Sims, Lauren Taylor MD, Richetta Wilkerson, Barbara Wyckoff, James Wyckoff, and Shelley Wyckoff.

We are especially grateful to Shannon Jones and Jamil Minnis for unconditional support through this process.

Thank you to all those whom have opened this book in the hopes to improve their wellbeing and health in a positive way.

ABOUT THE AUTHORS

Elita Wyckoff-Jones and Shamolie Wyckoff are siblings originally from Huntsville, Alabama. **Elita Wyckoff-Jones** is a practicing physician in Obstetrics and Gynecology for the past 15 years. She currently resides in Cary, North Carolina with her husband and two daughters. **Shamolie Wyckoff**, for the past 11 years, has been a practicing physician in Physical Medicine & Rehabilitation and Pain Medicine. She currently resides in Atlanta, Georgia.

Made in the USA
Coppell, TX
03 February 2021

49490953R00066